Pharmacy Technician Certification Exam

Miller's Essential Prep Study Guide For Passing the PTCE

Introduction

You're about to discover how to study and prepare for the Pharmacy Technician Certification Exam of the Pharmacy Technician Certification Board. You'll need it if you want to be prioritized when applying for a pharmacy technician job.

Through this study guide, you'll learn to focus on the following subjects and topics:

- ✓ Duties and responsibilities of the pharmacy technician;
- ✓ District and Federal laws and regulations governing controlled substances;
- ✓ District and Federal laws and regulations are governing the practice of pharmacy.
- ✓ Knowledge of prescription and non-prescription medications;
- ✓ Knowledge of drug therapy and its duration, routes of administration, physical appearance, dosage forms, and dose or strengths;
- ✓ Knowledge of special considerations for dosing geriatric and pediatric patients;
- ✓ The dispensing process;
- ✓ Pharmaceutical calculations;
- ✓ Requirements and professional standards for the:
    - o Preparation;
    - o Labeling;
    - o Dispensing;
    - o Storage;
    - o Prepackaging;
    - o Distribution; and

- o   Route of administration of medications;
- ✓ Sterile and non-sterile compounding;
- ✓ Drugs for the treatment of major chronic conditions;
- ✓ Interacting and communicating with patients;
- ✓ Confidentiality;
- ✓ Third party prescriptions;
- ✓ And more!

These areas will be your guide on what to study for the exam. There is also a mock exam at the end of this book that you can use to practice for your test. Correct answers are provided and explained after the test, so you can understand the reason for each correct answer.

Finally, you'll get to read some tips in this book on how you can prepare and study for the exam.

Thank you, and I hope you enjoy it!

© Copyright 2019 by Miller All rights reserved.

This document is geared towards providing exact and reliable information in regards to the topic and issue covered. The publication is sold with the idea that the publisher is not required to render accounting, officially permitted, or otherwise, qualified services. If advice is necessary, legal or professional, a practiced individual in the profession should be ordered.

- From a Declaration of Principles which was accepted and approved equally by a Committee of the American Bar Association and a Committee of Publishers and Associations.

In no way is it legal to reproduce, duplicate, or transmit any part of this document in either electronic means or in printed format. Recording of this publication is strictly prohibited, and any storage of this document is not allowed unless with written permission from the publisher. All rights reserved.

The information provided herein is stated to be truthful and consistent, in that any liability, in terms of inattention or otherwise, by any usage or abuse of any policies, processes, or directions contained within is the solitary and utter responsibility of the recipient reader. Under no circumstances will any legal responsibility or blame be held against the publisher for any reparation, damages, or monetary loss due to the information herein, either directly or indirectly.

Respective authors own all copyrights not held by the publisher.

The information herein is offered for informational purposes solely and is universal as so. The presentation of the information is without contract or any type of guarantee assurance.

PTCB was not involved in the creation or production of this product, is not in any way affiliated with Miller's Pharmacy Technician Exam Prep Team, and does not sponsor or endorse this product. All test names (and their acronyms) are trademarks of their respective owners. This study guide is for general information only and does not claim endorsement by any third party.

The trademarks that are used are without any consent, and the publication of the trademark is without permission or backing by the trademark owner. All trademarks and brands within this book are for clarifying purposes only and are the owned by the owners themselves, not affiliated with this document.

Table of Contents

The Basics_ CHAPTER 1

Pharmacy Technicians 14

    Job Description 14

Exam Background 16

    Job Analysis Study 16

    Updated Exam Blueprint 17

    Knowledge Domains and Areas 18

About the Exam 22

    Format and Content 22

    Scoring 22

    Applying for Certification 23

    Schedule the Exam 25

    Take the Pharmacy Technician Certification Exam 29

Exam Prep 30

    Official Pharmacy Technician Certification Board Practice Tools 30

Pharmacology for Technicians_CHAPTER 2

What is Pharmacology? 31

Generic and Brand Names of Drugs 32

Points to remember: 32

Therapeutic Equivalence..............................33

    Criteria 1: 33

    Criteria 2: 33

    Criteria 3: 33

    Criteria 4: 33

    Criteria 5: 33

Drug Interactions..34

    ✓   Drug-condition interactions:........................34

    ✓   Drug-food/beverage interactions 34

    ✓   Drug-drug interactions: 34

Pharmacotherapy..34

    Kinds of Drug Therapy...........................35

Drug Allergies, Contraindications, and Side Effects...35

Drug Dosage and Indication........................36

    Dosage Forms 36

Pharmacy Law and Regulations_CHAPTER 3

    General Scope of Laws and Regulations in Pharmacy 38

    Learning Objectives 39

Sterile and Non-Sterile Compounding_CHAPTER 4

Compounding 40

Compounding Pharmacy 41

Medication Safety_CHAPTER 5

Key Safety Checks 42

    Prescription Drop-Off 42

    Filling and Dispensing 42

    Order Entry 43

    Point of Sale 43

Pharmacy Quality Assurance_CHAPTER 6

Quality Assurance Activities 44

Quality and Safety 44

    1: 44

    2: 44

    3: 44

    4: 44

    Safe Working Environment 45

    Quality Products 45

    Risk Management and Quality Improvement 45

    Patient Safety Culture 46

Medication Order Entry and Fill Process_CHAPTER 7

The Script 47

Order Entry and Fill Process 47

Processing a Prescription 48

    Step 1: 48

    Step 2: 48

    Step 3: 48

    Step 4: 48

    Step 5: 48

Pharmacy Processing Key Points 48

Pharmacy Inventory Management_CHAPTER 8

Purpose and Goals of Inventory Management 50

    1: 51

    2: 51

    3: 51

    4: 51

Pharmacy Billing and Reimbursement_CHAPTER 9

Pharmacy Billing Cycle 52

Step 1: 52

Step 2: 52

Step 3: 52

Step 4: 52

Step 5: 52

Step 6: 52

Step 7: 52

Receiving a Patient's Prescription..............................52

Gathering Important Data from Patient 53

Data Entry 53

Pharmacy Claim Transmittal 54

Third-Party Payor Adjudication 54

Point-of-Sale 55

Payment Processing 55

Other Reimbursement Methods 55

  Episode-of-Care Reimbursement 55

  Fee-for-Service Reimbursement............................55

Pharmacy Information System Usage and Application_CHAPTER 10

Pharmacy Interfaces 56

  Pharmacy-centric: 56

Facility-centric: 57

Pharmacy Computer Applications 57

Practice Test_CHAPTER 11

Questions 59

Answers 64

The Basics_ CHAPTER 1

There are many opportunities available for pharmacy technicians in the United States. According to the Bureau of Labor Statistics (BLS) of the U.S. Department of Labor (DOL), there are 372,500 jobs (the latest available data is for the year 2014) for pharmacy technicians in the country. Majority of these jobs, around 75%, can be found in the pharmaceutical retail industry including online or mail-order drugstores, mass retailer chains (e.g., Walgreens), and independently-owned pharmacies. The remaining 25% work in pharmaceutical wholesalers, government-run agencies, and healthcare providers such as nursing homes and hospitals. You can take advantage of the job surplus, yet, you should meet certain prerequisite that may differ contingent upon the state where you live in or need to work in.

To work as a pharmacy technician and to be recognized as one, you must first be certified. You need to pass the Certification Exam administered by the Pharmacy Technician Certification Board. Through this exam, the board guarantees your competency and allows you to become a certified pharmacy technician.

Certification is useful to pharmacy technicians. It can help you administer medications properly and effortlessly. It enables you to handle patients that require medications. Most importantly, however, you will be prioritized to work alongside a licensed pharmacist if you hold a pharmacy technician certification.

Pharmacy Technicians

A certified pharmacy technician (CPhT) typically works in the healthcare industry. The job is directly supervised by a licensed or registered (or both) pharmacist in hospital, community, or retail pharmacies. However, it requires pharmacy-related functions not only in pharmacies, but in software companies, third-party insurance providers, drug manufacturers, and long-term healthcare facilities as well. Alternatively, a CPhT can work in colleges teaching pharmacology, pharmacotherapy, or other pharmaceutical-related subjects.

Job Description

Foremost, as a certified pharmacy technician, you will be dispensing prescription drugs to patients and instruct them on how to take their medications. In other cases, you will also provide them with medical devices they need and teach them how to use such instruments properly. You will also answer patient inquiries or arrange for them to speak to a pharmacist if they have concerns about their medications.

You are also expected to perform administrative duties including encoding patients' medical records, reviewing prescriptions, collecting patients' information, organizing an inventory of drugs, processing insurance claims, and taking phone inquiries from customers. You will also carry out cashier and other over-the-counter (OTC) duties such as using the cash register and accepting payment for purchased medications. In general, you have to make sure that customers get the right medications they need, are informed of how to take their medicines or use their medical devices, and accept payments for purchased items.

In healthcare facilities, you will also pack and dispense drugs in satellite pharmacies, but instead of giving them directly to patients, you will distribute them to nursing units. You are also expected to use the aseptic technique to mix intravenous medications. You will also perform administrative duties such as documenting drug inventory and patients' medical records.

In recent years, the shortage of pharmacists has amplified the need for more well-trained, certified pharmacy technicians. Because of this, the duties and responsibilities of pharmacy technicians have increased including infection control, pharmacotherapeutics, and alternative medicine.

Considering the responsibilities you'll face, the Board of Pharmacy in each US state implements strict educational and certification requirements. For example, a state may hire you only if you received the proper education and training for pharmacy technicians, are registered with the Division of Professional Regulation, and certified by the Pharmacy Technician Certification Board.

The educational requirement includes a high school diploma with work training, an associate degree, or technical school education. If you have accomplished any of the three, you can take the Pharmacy Technician Certification Exam. It was developed as a gauge to determine if those who finished the educational requirements for pharmacy technicians can properly practice and demonstrate what they have learned from school and training.

Exam Background

The Pharmacy Technician Certification Exam is a national certification exam developed based on the Job Analysis Study.

Job Analysis Study

The Job Analysis Study is a regularly-conducted study by the Pharmacy Technician Certification Board. It serves as the foundation for the exam that the board administers to implement its accreditation standards and industry best practices. The most recent study, conducted from August 2011 to January 2012, was aided by American College Testing, Inc. (ACT), a standard in college-readiness assessment for admission in the US and other Canadian colleges and universities. ACT and the board worked closely with Subject Matter Experts (SMEs) in the field of pharmacy.

The study's purpose was to evaluate and determine the required knowledge to fulfill the job of a pharmacy technician. It was designed to gather data on the skills, tasks, and knowledge areas of the occupation in all practice settings and states. Information collected was then used to develop a test outline (or as the board calls it, test blueprint) to be used for the Pharmacy Technician Certification Exam.

There were three phases that comprised the study:

> **Phase 1:** Two survey instruments were developed. The first survey inquired the tasks that pharmacy technicians perform, the tasks' importance, and the tasks' frequency on a daily

basis. The second survey helped identify the skills and knowledge needed to accomplish the pharmacy technician's tasks.

Phase 2: The surveys were distributed, collected, and analyzed. There were 25,712 pharmacy technicians from all practice settings (e.g., military, hospital, community) and states who participated in the surveys.

Phase 3: The panel of SMEs used the resulting survey data to develop the blueprint for the Pharmacy Technician Certification Exam. The blueprint focused primarily on the skills and knowledge linked to the frequent and most important tasks performed by pharmacy technicians. It was then forwarded to the Certification Council and Board of Governors of the Pharmacy Technician Certification Board for final approval.

The first Pharmacy Technician Certification Exam blueprint was released in February 2012.

Updated Exam Blueprint

However, the Certification Council and Board of Governors of the Pharmacy Technician Certification Board updated the 2012 Job Analysis Study and released an updated test blueprint on November 2013. You have to familiarize yourself with the changes made in the blueprint to make sure that you are using the right resources and materials when reviewing for the exam.

To help those familiar with the old test to understand the changes in the new version, the Pharmacy Technician Certification Board provided a crosswalk. It identifies knowledge areas that were added to the new Pharmacy Technician Certification Exam blueprint. For more details about the update, please visit the Crosswalk Between Old PTCE Knowledge Statements and Current Knowledge Areas on the board's website.

Knowledge Domains and Areas

There are nine knowledge domains included in the updated test blueprint for the Pharmacy Technician Certification Exam. Each one has been scrutinized by the board and was deemed critical to the pharmacy technician practice. Each domain also includes sub-domains or knowledge areas:

Domain	Area	Content
1.0 Pharmacology for Technicians		13.75%
	1.1 Generic & brand names of pharmaceuticals	
	1.2 Therapeutic equivalence	
	1.3 Drug interactions	
	1.4 Drug therapy	
	1.5 Common and severe drug side effects, contraindications, and allergies	
	1.6 Medications, herbal, and dietary supplements dosage and indication	
2.0 Pharmacy Law and Regulations		12.50%
	2.1 Disposal, handling, and storage of hazardous wastes and substances	
	2.2 Hazardous substances treatment, prevention, and exposure	
	2.3 Transfer regulations for controlled substances	

2.4 Documentation requirements (e.g., ordering, receiving, returning, destruction, loss/theft) for controlled substances

2.5 Formula used to verify the validity of a prescriber's Drug Enforcement Agency (DEA) number

2.6 Record documentation, keeping, and retention

2.7 Programs for restricted drugs and related requirements for prescription-processing

2.8 Professional standards related to data confidentiality, security, and integrity

2.9 Requirement for consultation

2.10 FDA's recall classification

2.11 Standards for infection control

2.12 Recordkeeping for recalled and repackaged supplies and products

2.13 Professional standards on the responsibilities and roles of pharmacy technicians, pharmacists, and other employees in pharmacies

2.14 Reconciliation between federal and state laws and regulations

2.15 Supply, equipment, and facility requirements

3.0 Sterile and Non-Sterile Compounding — 8.75%

3.1 Infection control

3.2 Handling and disposal requirements

3.3 Compounding record, batch preparation, and other documentation

3.4 Determining product stability

3.5 Selection and use of supplies

and equipment
3.6 Sterile compounding processes
3.7 Non-sterile compounding processes

4.0 Medication Safety — 12.50%

4.1 Error prevention strategies for data entry
4.2 Medication guide and patient package insert requirements
4.3 Identify issues that require pharmacist intervention
4.4 Look-alike/sound-alike medications
4.5 High-alert/risk medications
4.6 Common safety strategies

5.0 Pharmacy Quality Assurance — 7.50%

5.1 Inventory control systems and quality assurance practices
5.2 Infection control documentation and procedures
5.3 Regulations and guidelines of risk management
5.4 Necessary communication channels to ensure appropriate problem follow-up and resolution
5.5 Efficiency, customer satisfaction, and productivity measures

6.0 Medication Order Entry and Fill Process — 17.50%

6.1 Order entry process
6.2 Data entry, intake, and interpretation
6.3 Calculate doses required
6.4 Fill process

6.5 Labeling requirements
6.6 Packaging requirements
6.7 Dispensing process

7.0 Pharmacy Inventory Management — 8.75%

7.1 Function and application of National Drug Code (NDC), expiration dates, and lot numbers
7.2 Approved/preferred or formulary product list
7.3 Ordering and receiving processes
7.4 Storage requirements
7.5 Removal of inventory

8.0 Pharmacy Billing and Reimbursement — 8.75%

8.1 Reimbursement plans and policies
8.2 Third-party resolution
8.3 Third-party reimbursement systems
8.4 Healthcare reimbursement systems
8.5 Coordination of benefits

9.0 Pharmacy Information System Usage and Application — 10%

9.1 Computer applications for pharmacy-related tasks especially for the documentation of the dispensing of medication orders or prescriptions
9.2 Documentation management, pharmacy computer applications, and databases

For the full, updated blueprint, please visit the Pharmacy Technician Certification Exam Blueprint. You will learn all you need to study for from each knowledge area of the exam.

About the Exam

Format and Content

The Pharmacy Technician Certification Exam is a two-hour, computer-based exam. You will be answering 90 multiple-choice questions with 80 of which are scored while the remaining unscored items contain a survey and exam tutorial. You have to finish the scored questions within 1 hour and 50 minutes, while the unscored items should be finished within 10 minutes.

There are four conceivable responses for each inquiry and just a single right answer. Your score is determined based on the correct responses you've provided for the 80 scored items.

Scoring

Passing Score and Rates

To pass the test, you'll need a scaled passing score of 1400. Since the exam was first implemented in 1995 until December 2016, the passing rate for the test is 72%. To date, there have been 618,408 pharmacy technician certifications that the board has granted to individuals.

Hand Scoring

If you failed the exam, but want your scaled score to be further examined, you can have it verified by manual review or hand, which is called hand scoring. You must fill out a Hand Score Request

Form and submit it to the board within 30 days after you received your scaled score. You will be paying $50 for the processing of your request.

In any case, note that the board's decision is final once the hand score is uncovered. At the same time, the board has never changed; in its history, a scaled score based on the result of manual reviewing.

Confidentiality of Scores Policy

The Pharmacy Technician Certification Board has the right to provide proof whether or not you are currently certified to any organization or person who requests the information.

Applying for Certification

Eligibility

To be a certified pharmacy technician, you should fulfill the following requirements:

- ✓ Accomplish a passing score on the Pharmacy Technician Certification Exam.

- ✓ Compliance with all of the certification policies of the Pharmacy Technician Certification Board.

- ✓ Full disclosure of State Board of Pharmacy registration, licensure, and all criminal actions and records against you.

- ✓ High school or equivalent educational diploma (e.g., Certificate of High School Equivalency or GED).

However, you may be disqualified for certification if the board discovers:

- You have a criminal record;
- You have received disciplinary actions from the State Board of Pharmacy registration and licensure offices even during and after receiving the certification;
- You have violated a certification policy, especially the board's Code of Conduct.

The Pharmacy Technician Certification Board reserves the right to verify eligibility, investigate criminal record, and deny certification to any applicant of its certification.

Submitting an Application

Submitting an application for certification can only be done online. You should go on the board's website and register for an account first. Subsequent to confirming your email address, you would now be able to apply for accreditation.

Upon applying for a certification, you have 30 days to submit supporting documents required by the board. If you neglect to finish all necessities inside this period, the board will refund your payment but will deduct $25 for administrative fees.

The initial cost of the Pharmacy Technician Certification Exam is only $129. If you failed the test and would want to take another one, you will only pay $40.

Testing Accommodations for Individuals with Disabilities

The paper application is also available, but it is only reserved for individuals with disabilities or those who find it hard to apply online. However, a written request for this type of application should be first sent to the board. The request must include appropriate documentation of the individual's hardship or disability.

The same applies to those requesting for testing accommodations. The board will provide individuals with accommodations consistent with the American with Disabilities Act (ADA) at no additional cost. However, if medical equipment used by a person with a disability is not listed in the allowed items for the exam, it should be approved by the board first. The individual involved will yet again, send a written request for the accommodation of the medical equipment in concern.

Schedule the Exam

Authorization Period

Once your registration and application have been successful, you still can't set a schedule for your exam. You have to wait for an email that the board will send to you. It contains an authorized time frame on when you can properly schedule an exam appointment. Once you receive this email, you have 90 days to finalize your test schedule.

Withdrawing an Application

If you want to cancel your application, or you were not able to finalize a test scheduled within the 90-day period, you can withdraw from the test using your Pharmacy Technician Certification Board account. You will get a refund, but the board will charge you a minimum of $25 for administrative fees.

Scheduling

The Pharmacy Technician Certification Exam is held in over 350 professional centers of Pearson Education Inc.., otherwise known as Pearson VUE (Virtual University Enterprise), all over the US.

To schedule your exam appointment, you have two options. You can set your schedule online at http://www.pearsonvue.com/ptcb/ using your Pharmacy Technician Certification Board account. You can also schedule your exam with Pearson VUE through phone at (866) 902-0593. Individuals who have requested a testing accommodation can schedule their exam through a different number at (800) 466-0450.

Pearson VUE will send a confirmation email within 24 hours of the successful scheduled exam. Once you've confirmed your appointment, you are now set for the exam.

Canceling & Rescheduling

You have to email or call Pearson VUE at least 24 hours before your scheduled appointment. You will not have to pay or cancellation or rescheduling of your exam.

Missed Appointments

However, if you missed your appointment, all fees you have paid will be forfeited. If the reason for your absence was an emergency though, you could file for an emergency withdrawal request with the board. Situations or incidences considered emergencies are:

- Serious illness
- Court appearance
- Serious accident
- Death in the immediate family
- Unexpected hospitalization
- Injury

An emergency should've happened on the day of your exam to be considered by the board for withdrawal. You must submit proof of your emergency situation along with an Emergency Withdrawal Request form to the board for approval.

Take the Pharmacy Technician Certification Exam

Before the Exam

Don't forget to confirm your appointment. Arrive 30 minutes before your appointment on the day of the exam. Bring with you an ID that should match the name you entered in your Pharmacy Technician Certification Board account. With an approved form of ID, you will not be allowed to take the test. Here are the accepted forms of ID you can bring:

- ✓
- ✓ Government-Issued Driving Learner's Permit
- ✓ Government-Issued Driver's License
- ✓ Passport/Passport Card
- ✓ Military ID
- ✓ US Department of Homeland Security-Issued Employment Authorization Card
- ✓ Permanent Resident Card (Green Card)

If any of the above IDs don't have a photo and signature, you can present secondary IDs such as the following:

- ✓ Employee/School ID

- ✓ ATM/Debit Card
- ✓ Credit Card
- ✓ Social Security Card

All IDs must still be valid or unexpired, and with a clear photo and signature.

Please take note that calculators are not allowed in the testing room. A calculator is already provided within the exam. However, if you prefer a physical calculator, you may request from a test center staff or proctor.

During the Exam

During the exam, you are expected to adhere to the Pharmacy Technician Certification Board's candidate attestation, test center rules, and Code of Conduct. An agreement including these terms and conditions are presented before you proceed with the exam. You should accept the agreement to start the test. You are also expected to complete the pre-test tutorial after accepting the agreement.

After the Exam

After the examination, you will be asked to answer a brief survey. An unofficial score will be presented on your screen after taking the survey. It will be printed and handed over to you. You will receive the official result within two to three weeks, and it will be posted on your Pharmacy Technician Certification Board account, after which your certificate will be made available for printing.

Retake Policy

You could retake the test after 60 days since receiving your test results. However, this is only applicable to the second and third attempts. For your fourth attempt, you will have to wait 6 months to be allowed to take the test again. On your fifth and following attempts, you will have to provide written proof to the board that you have done all your best to review the knowledge domains and areas that are included in the test. The board will accept the following preparation activities:

- ✓ Graduation from an (A.S.) program
- ✓ Completion of an ASHP/ACPE-accredited training program
- ✓

The Pharmacy Technician Certification Board encourages applicants to prepare thoroughly for the exam, especially if you're retaking it. According to the board, if you failed the exam once, there's a high chance you'll fail the succeeding tests that's why it's important to be always prepared.

Exam Prep

You can prepare for the exam using tutorials and practice tests from different sources. Just make sure that the topics you are studying and reviewing are included in the updated version of the certification test.

The Pharmacy Certification Technician Board and Pearson VUE also have tutorials and practice tools that you can take advantage of.

Official Pharmacy Technician Certification Board Practice Tools

The Pharmacy Certification Technician Board features two practice tools:

The Official Pharmacy Certification Technician Board Calculations Practice Questions App: the app is available for iOS and Android mobile devices.

The Updated Official Pharmacy Certification Technician Board Practice Exam: you have to create a separate Pharmacy Certification Technician Board account to avail of the practice test, which is worth $29. Like the real deal, it includes 90 questions that you have to finish within 2 hours.

Pharmacology for Technicians_CHAPTER 2

The first knowledge area of the test, the Pharmacology for Technicians, covers 13.75% of the entire Pharmacy Technician Certification Exam. Over the years, pharmacology has evolved to the extent that it is now used to study the biological effects of drugs. It was originally used to describe what biologically active chemicals can do, but it has expanded from that beginning. Now let's briefly explore this scientific study that is important for pharmacy technicians.

What is Pharmacology?

In the broadest sense, the study of pharmacology involves the effects of natural and synthetic chemical agents on biological systems. To determine these effects, different aspects of the use of therapeutic and non-therapeutic drugs are studied. This includes biological transformations, mechanisms of action, behavioral and physiological effects, chemical properties, and derivation of different kinds of chemical agents. As a result, pharmacology is used to

- ✓ determine the effects of chemical agents upon physiological or behavioral, systemic, and subcellular processes;
- ✓ deal with the dangers of herbicides and pesticides ;
- ✓ or focus on the prevention and treatment of diseases.

Pharmacology incorporates skills and knowledge from several science disciplines; that's why it is often depicted as a bridge science. It involves molecular and cell biology, biochemistry, and physiology. These disciplines are used to develop therapeutics in pharmacology.

For this area of the exam, you need to study the following topics:

- ✓ Generic and brand names of pharmaceuticals
- ✓ Therapeutic equivalence
- ✓ Drug interactions: e.g., drug-disease, drug-drug, drug-dietary supplement, drug-OTC, drug-laboratory, drug-nutrient
- ✓ Drug therapy: e.g., strengths/dose, dosage forms, physical appearance, routes of administration, and duration of drug therapy
- ✓ Allergies, contraindications, and side effects associated with medications
- ✓ Medications, herbal, and dietary supplements dosage and indication

To better understand each area of the exam, here's a brief description of what you should be studying about (1.0) Pharmacology.

Generic and Brand Names of Drugs

Drugs are often given several names. At first, it is given a chemical name upon its first discovery. This name describes the molecular or atomic structure of the drug. However, the chemical name is usually long, too complex, and hard to remember for general and public use. A shorthand version is thus developed. It is typically a code name given to a drug such as 71 CIBA for Serap-ES, an antihypertensive drug manufactured by Novartis Pharmaceuticals. This shorthand version is used by researchers for easy referencing.

Still, code names are too complex for public use. United States Adopted Names Council (USAN Council) assigns unique generic names for drugs as soon as the (FDA) approves them for safe and effective use. At the same time, the manufacturer provides a brand name for their drugs.

The generic name is the official name of drugs that you see in pharmacies, while the brand name is the trademark or propriety name owned by the manufacturers. Brand names are especially used when a drug is protected by a patent. However, either the generic or brand names may be used by a manufacturer if they want to sell an off-patent drug as long as they secure permission to sell drugs that are no longer patent protected.

Compared to brand names, generic names are more difficult to remember; that's why it's important for you to study the most common generic and brand names.

Points to remember:

✓ A generic name is a shortened version of a drug's formula, structure, and chemical name. For example:

Generic Name and (Brand Name)	Chemical Name
Acetaminophen and hydrocodone (Vicodin)	4,5α-epoxy-3-methoxy-17-methylmorphinan-6-one tartrate (1:1) hydrate (2:5)

33

Atorvastatin (Lipitor)	(3R,5R)-7-[2-(4-fluorophenyl)-3-phenyl-4-(phenylcarbamoyl)-5-propan-2-ylpyrrol-1-yl]-3,5-dihydroxyheptanoic acid
Oxymetazoline (Visine)	3-[(4,5-dihydro-1H-imidazole-2-yl)methyl]-6-(1,1-dimethylethyl)-2,4-dimethyl-phenol hydrochloride

- ✓ A brand name, on the other hand, is often easy to remember, catchy, related to the intended purpose of a drug, or simply its shortened version. For example:

Generic Name	Brand Name
Minocycline	Minocin (a shortened version of its generic name)
Glipizide	Glucotrol (controls glucose, or blood sugar, levels)
Metoprolol	Lopressor (keeps blood pressure low or normal)

- ✓ Generic drugs are usually available at a lower cost compared to branded drugs even if it is manufactured by big brands. However, this doesn't mean that its efficiency, value, and standards are compromised. These drugs receive the same evaluation and requirements that branded names do. Customers, however, may prefer one drug to another because of varied reasons.

Therapeutic Equivalence

Drugs are considered to have therapeutic equivalence if they have the same safety profile and clinical effect when used by patients following a specified condition indicated in the labeling. In this topic, you need to study the therapeutic equivalence of certain drugs.

To determine if a drug is the therapeutic equivalence of another drug, FDA provided a number of criteria:

Criteria 1: it had complied with the Current Good Manufacturing Practice Regulations when it was manufactured

Criteria 2: it has been labeled adequately

Criteria 3: it is bioequivalent meaning:

a: it meets a suitable in vitro standard

b: it doesn't present a potential or known bioequivalence problem

c: if it does present a problem, it should comply with a proper bioequivalence standard

Criteria 4: it has the same pharmaceutical effect based on:

a: applicable standards of identity, purity, quality, and strength

b: equivalent amounts of the same active ingredient

c: the same dosage and form of drug administration (e.g., orally, intravenously, topical, intramuscular, or sublingual)

Criteria 5: it was approved effective and safe by FDA

If certain drugs meet the criteria above, they are considered therapeutically equivalent by the FDA regardless of:

- ✓ physical characteristics
- ✓ storage conditions
- ✓ minor labeling aspects (e.g., pharmacokinetic information)
- ✓ expiration time or date
- ✓ excipients (inactive substances including preservatives, flavors, and colors, that serve as a vehicle for other active substances or drugs)
- ✓ packaging
- ✓ release mechanisms, and
- ✓ scoring configuration.

Drug Interactions

Doctors need to understand if a patient is taking several medicines at a time. This helps avoid problems that drug interactions can cause such as increased action, unexpected side effects, or decreased efficiency. Drugs interact differently with a patient's dietary supplements, over-the-counter drugs, laboratory procedures or diagnostics, and even nutrients in the body. In general,, however, drug interaction has three categories:

- ✓ **Drug-condition interactions:** occurs when certain drugs react with an existing medical condition. For example, if you have liver disease, you could experience worsening health or unwanted health reactions if you take certain antibiotics, anticonvulsants, antidepressants, antifungal drugs, and more.

- ✓ **Drug-food/beverage interactions** occur when certain drugs react with foods or beverages. For example, mixing alcohol with certain medications may cause harmful effects to your health, even death.

- ✓ **Drug-drug interactions:** occur when drugs react with other medications. Often, drug-drug interaction causes unexpected, harmful side effects. For example, sedatives and antihistamine (for allergies) shouldn't be taken together when a patient will operate heavy machinery or drive a car. When taken together, these drugs can impair a person's senses and make certain situations dangerous.

Pharmacy technicians are expected to inform patients of the various drug interactions that may occur based on the categories mentioned above. You should also be studying the information provided in drug labels that you can relay to patients buying drugs from you. Such information includes:

- ✓ what is a drug's intended use
- ✓ how to take it

- ✓ how to reduce the risk of potentially harmful drug interactions

Pharmacotherapy

With pharmacotherapy or drug therapy, you'll be studying about the effects of the duration, routes of administration, physical appearance, dosage forms, dose, and strengths of drugs while it is being used to treat diseases. To cure or reduce illnesses and promote healthy function of cells, medications are used to interact with enzymes and receptors. It is researched and then tested thoroughly before it is prescribed to or used on patients. However, specific effects brought about by other drugs, dietary supplements, herbal remedies, or certain foods may have been unanticipated in the process. Pharmacotherapy studies these kinds of stuff.

Pharmacists are experts in drug therapy. They are responsible for the commercial, appropriate, and safe use of pharmaceutical drugs. Because you'll be working alongside a pharmacist, it's also important for you to understand pharmacotherapy. As part of your responsibility, you'll be directly providing patient care, act as the main source of information about medications, and even work as a part of a multidisciplinary team of healthcare professionals. To function well in your position, you'll require skills, experience, training, and knowledge in clinical, pharmaceutical, and biomedical sciences.

Kinds of Drug Therapy

Medications can treat many medical conditions. Illnesses that cannot be cured can even be improved by pharmacotherapy as it eliminates symptoms experienced by a patient. Here are some examples of drug therapy you should study further for your exam:

- ✓ Antidepressants to reduce symptoms of depression

- ✓ Long- or short-term medication to fight drug dependence and addiction

- ✓ Pain relief following an accident or surgery

- ✓ Antibiotics to treat common ailments

Drug Allergies, Contraindications, and Side Effects

In this section of the test, you'll be demonstrating your skills and knowledge of side effects, contradictions, adverse effects, and allergies of medications to:

- ✓ Provide patient with information about the potential interactions, adverse effects, and common side effects of medications

- ✓ Inform a patient when the primary healthcare provider should be notified in case of interactions, adverse effects, and common side effects of medications

- ✓

- ✓ Document interactions, adverse effects, and common side effects of medications and drug therapy

- ✓ Document and evaluate a patient's response and actions taken to counteract interactions, adverse effects, and common side effects of medications and drug therapy

- ✓ Identify the evidence and symptoms of an allergic reaction to medications

- ✓ Identify potential and actual incompatibilities of prescribed medications

- ✓ Identify a contraindication to the route of administration of a medication

Pharmacy technicians must be knowledgeable about the interactions, adverse effects, side effects, indications, contraindication, and allergies associated with medications when they are ordered. If your knowledge of patients' medical records is not congruent and consistent with patients' conditions, you are in the position to discuss these concerns with the doctors or licensed practitioners who ordered or prescribed the drugs.

Drug Dosage and Indication

Aside from patient education about adverse effects, side effects, contraindications, and allergies associated with drugs, you are expected to provide complete information about the medications that a patient has to take. You should be providing the following information at the least about a medication:

- ✓ name and purpose
- ✓ dosage
- ✓ when and how often it should be taken
- ✓ special instructions like taking a medication 30 minutes before a meal
- ✓ indications and contraindications
- ✓ possible side effects including its signs and symptoms
- ✓ possible adverse effects including its signs and symptoms
- ✓ drug interactions with other medications, supplements, foods, and beverages

Because you'll be providing this information, you should be familiar with the dosage and indication of legend, dietary and herbal supplements, OTC medications, and other common forms of medications. Here's a summary of what you have to be prepared about:

Dosage Forms

Here are the most common forms of dosages that can be given to patients. Each form has its own routes of administrations.

Enteral drugs: passes through the gastrointestinal (GI) tract, absorbed into the blood, and metabolized by the liver. This includes

- ✓ oral,
- ✓ rectal, and
- ✓ nasogastric routes.

Parenteral medicines: refers to injections in general pharmacy. This includes routes of administrations through

- ✓ inhalation,
- ✓ topical and
- ✓ injection.

While topical and inhalation routes are included under this form of drug dosage, the two are distinct and have their own routes of administration.

Topical medications: applied to a mucous membrane or the skin surface.

Inhaled drugs: are inhaled through the nose or mouth. This type of drugs is often used for the treatment of respiratory diseases. In other cases, however, inhaled drugs are used for general anesthesia.

Injectable medications: typically in the form of powders or solutions that are diluted in a sterile diluent to create a compound injectable solution.

The most common dosage forms are oral and injectable medication. These two are available in many forms of preparations such as the ones in the table below:

Oral Preparations (Enteral Form)	**Injectable Preparations (Parenteral Form)**
✓ Tablets: chewable, sublingual (placed under the tongue), film coated, wafers (placed on the tongue), enteric coated, controlled release, slow release, fast acting, and buccal (placed between the gums and cheek) tablets. ✓ Capsules: medications encased in an oval-shaped shell or gelatin form ✓ Caplet: oval-shaped tablets ✓ Lozenge and troche: left in the mouth to melt. ✓ Oral solutions: drug is completely mixed with liquid ✓ Oral suspensions: drug is partially mixed with liquid.	✓ Intravenous (IV): injected into the vein. The most common form is the IV drip or infusion. ✓ Epidural: injected into the epidural space of the spinal cord. ✓ ✓ Intramuscular: injected into the muscle ✓ Intra-articular: injected into the joint ✓ Intraocular : injected within the eye ✓ Intracardiac: injected into the heart

Should be shaken before administered to the patient.
- ✓ Oral powders: dissolved in water or juice before administered to a patient
- ✓ Syrups: contains sugar or sucrose
- ✓ Emulsions: two forms of liquid that don't mix well
- ✓ Elixirs: contains 5%-40% alcohol
- ✓ Tinctures: contains 17%-80% alcohol
- ✓ Inhalation

Pharmacy Law and Regulations_CHAPTER 3

Pharmacy law and regulations make up 12.50% of the exam. It is divided into the following areas:

1. Disposal, handling, and storage of hazardous wastes and substances
2. Hazardous substances treatment, prevention, and exposure
3. Transfer regulations for controlled substances
4. Documentation requirements (e.g., ordering, receiving, returning, destruction, loss/theft) for controlled substances
5. The formula used to verify the validity of a prescriber's Drug Enforcement Agency (DEA) number
6. Record documentation, keeping, and retention
7. Programs for restricted drugs and related requirements for prescription-processing
8. Professional standards related to data confidentiality, security, and integrity
9. Requirement for consultation
10. FDA's recall classification
11. Standards for infection control
12. Record keeping for recalled and repackaged supplies and products
13. Professional standards on the responsibilities and roles of pharmacy technicians, pharmacists, and other employees in pharmacies
14. Reconciliation between federal and state laws and regulations

15. Supply, equipment, and facility requirements

General Scope of Laws and Regulations in Pharmacy

The implementation of laws to regulate professions in the pharmacy industry is broad and wide. Every aspect is virtually governed including disciplinary actions, prohibited conduct, requirements for dispensing prescriptions, the scope of practice, pharmacy licensure requirements, and even employment of pharmacy technicians. Although pharmacy laws are generally similar between states, specific requirements still vary. The state Board of Pharmacy handles violations of pharmacy laws, including ones made by pharmacy technicians.

Laws are created through different means. State administrative agencies such as the Board of Pharmacy in each state adopt regulations. Laws, on the other hand, are enacted by state legislatures or the US Congress. Laws about the permitted duties and requirements for licensure or registration of pharmacy technicians are applied in many states. However, because of the varying laws and regulations between states, it would be advantageous for pharmacy technicians to be familiar with local pharmacy laws.

Pharmacy technicians are also subject to the profession's ethical principles and practice standards. Ethical principles provide a moral and ethical framework for the delivery of pharmacy care that technicians should provide. Practice standards meanwhile, provide a guide for the performance of pharmacy services.

Learning Objectives

Your learning objectives for this topic include the following:

1. Identify the different legal systems involved when a legal dispute is faced for a violation of any of the pharmacy laws and/or regulations.

2. Identify the processes that should be applied to establish ethical principles, professional practice standards, regulations, and laws.

3. Understand the impact of ethical principles and professional standards to the pharmacy technician practice.

4. Identify the role and purpose of laws, regulations, and rules in pharmacy

5. Identify differences between ethical principles and professional practice standards, and laws and regulations in pharmacy

Your sources of information for these objectives are:

- ✓ Federal laws and regulations
- ✓ State laws and regulations
- ✓ Professional practice standards
- ✓ Ethical principles
- ✓ Case law

Pharmacy technician students and those who are in training often wonder over the strict oversight or supervision of the pharmacy industry and profession. Your roles and responsibilities as a technician are the most obvious reasons.

While working under the supervision of a pharmacist, you'll be responsible for delivering drugs and pharmacotherapy-related services in various settings and healthcare sites including long-term care facilities, hospitals, and community pharmacies. You'll oversee the provision of medications to all members of society. You will also provide information about various drugs not only to patients but also to varying levels of healthcare professionals. You will assist and provide counsel to patients about their drug therapy. You will also assist them in selecting the right OTC medications for their ailments.

With pharmacy laws and regulations, you will be able to safely and effectively deliver products and services.

Sterile and Non-Sterile Compounding_CHAPTER 4

The domain of sterile and non-sterile compounding makes up 8.75% of the exam. Here are the knowledge areas that you need to study about under this domain:

1. Infection control
2. Handling and disposal requirements
3. Compounding record, batch preparation, and other documentation
4. Determining product stability
5. Selection and use of supplies and equipment
6. Sterile compounding processes
7. Non-sterile compounding processes

Compounding

According to the U.S. Pharmacopeia Convention (USP), compounding involves the preparation, mixture, assembly, alteration, labeling, and packaging of drugs. The whole process should follow the medication order or prescription. In some cases, the initiative of the pharmacist or pharmacy technician can be considered or accepted based on the professional relationship with a compounder or patient.

In general, however, compounding is defined as the creation of a drug or pharmaceutical preparation by a licensed pharmacist or certified pharmacy technician. This is done based on the following reasons:

- ✓ a patient requires a drug that was discontinued or is currently in shortage.

- ✓ a patient requires a drug with a specified preparation that is not commercially available

- ✓ . A patient can't tolerate a required drug that is sold in pharmacies or

- ✓ to meet a patient's unique requirements when a commercial drug can't meet those needs.

On the other hand, here are some examples of how pharmacy technicians compound medications to meet patients' needs or follow a doctor's prescription:

- ✓ Change the form of medication because patients are experiencing an upset stomach or having difficulty swallowing an oral medication.

- ✓ Reformulate a drug to remove nonessential, unwanted ingredients to which patients are allergic to. Examples of such ingredients include dye, gluten, and lactose.

- ✓ Give a medication a pleasant taste or add flavor to it, so children can easily take it orally.

- ✓ Customize a drug's dosage or strength.

Compounding allows pharmacy technicians to add drugs into different dosage forms including suppositories, transdermal gels, topical creams, and specially flavored liquids to suit patients' needs. However, it doesn't involve reproducing commercial drugs, which is against the law. Pharmaceutical compounding is entirely different from the commercial manufacturing of drugs.

Drug manufacturing involves mass producing drugs approved by the FDA. Products are then sold to healthcare facilities, medical professionals, and of course, pharmacies. They can also be sold in Stores authorized to resell by the government can also order commercially manufactured drugs.

Pharmaceutical compounding, on the other hand, is a traditional process of preparing medications to meet the exact specifications of a doctor. The resulting compound is directly dispensed to the requesting patient. It is performed by a pharmacy technician and supervised by a licensed pharmacist, although pharmacists can also do the compounding.

Compounding Pharmacy

Many pharmacies provide some level of compounding services. There are, however, pharmacies that focus mainly on compounding. According to the American Pharmacists Association, there are only 7,500 pharmacies that offer compounding services in the US. That's out of 56,000 pharmacies operating in various communities.

Compounding pharmacies invest in training and equipment to provide a more effective and safe compounding. They offer preparations that can be non-sterile or sterile. Below is a table of examples for each type of compounding preparations.

Sterile	Non-Sterile
✓ Eye medications ✓ Injection for the blood or body tissues	✓ Capsules ✓ Liquids ✓ Creams ✓ Ointments ✓ Other forms used in body areas where it is not necessary for medications to be absolutely sterile

Compounding pharmacies are easy to identify. You'll know one if you see compounding tools such as:

- ✓ ointment slabs for compounding creams and other skin preparations
- ✓ spatulas for mixing materials
- ✓ balances for weighing solids
- ✓ graduated cylinders for measuring liquids
- ✓ mortar and pestle for grinding materials

Compounding is a fundamental part of a pharmacy technician's practice. As part of the process of compounding, you will be responsible for the identification and preparation of the correct ingredients. You will be making sure that finished products and ingredients are free of physical contaminants and impurities such as chemical contaminants and precipitates. You will also test and ensure the compatibility, stability, and strength of compounded drugs. Of course, you will also have to package compounded medications and label them accurately before dispensing to patients.

Medication Safety_CHAPTER 5

Medication Safety makes up 12.50% of the exam. It is divided into the following areas:

1. Error prevention strategies for data entry
2. Medication guide and patient package insert requirements
3. Identify issues that require pharmacist intervention
4. Look-alike/sound-alike medications
5. High-alert/risk medications
6. Common safety strategies

While pharmacists play a major role in the modern practice of pharmacy, they rely on pharmacy technicians to provide an extra layer of medication safety. This is the reason why it's vital for technicians to adhere to system-based processes. As part of medication safety, technicians are expected to coordinate with pharmacists regarding their concerns and questions about processes that they believe are unmanageable or inefficient.

Key Safety Checks

Pharmacy technicians assist pharmacists, in all types of pharmacy settings, in performing different kinds of medication safety checks. Here are the key areas and production processes that technicians must provide added medication safety procedures for patients and customers.

Prescription Drop-Off

As a pharmacy technician, you'll be stationed at the prescription drop-off most of the time. While there, it would be your job to create a checklist of patient information that is critical to providing the right medications and service. You will be tasked with obtaining patient information as well in order to accomplish the contents of the checklist.

Patient information, such as date of birth, is used by pharmacists as a second identifier for patients. This is important for verification purposes, making it imperative to provide such personal information on every prescription hard copy. Other important information such as medical conditions (e.g., diabetes, pregnancy) and allergy must be updated in the patient profile whenever a patient visits the pharmacy to purchase medications. These updates should be relayed to the pharmacist for verification. This personal medical information help pharmacists verify if prescriptions are written for the wrong drug or incorrectly.

Filling and Dispensing

Incorrectly reading a label often results in many mix-ups during filling and dispensing. It's a problem made worse and motivated by confirmation bias. This occurs when pharmacy technicians or pharmacists select medications that are expected or familiar based on patient information, rather than providing drugs that are actually written on the prescription.

A pharmacy technician, for example, may choose a medication based on a mental recollection of the drug. Some of the most common mistakes occur when technicians rely on the characteristics of a drug – it may be the label, color, size, or shape, of the drug. Sometimes, the wrong drug is selected from the shelf without properly reading the label because the right medication was previously located on that same spot. Even the right container can be subject to confirmation bias. As a consequence, the wrong product is picked up and dispensed.

There are two typical solutions to these problems. Pharmacy technicians, while they are mostly expected to conduct inventory, should separate and label drugs that look alike. The use of technology, such as scanned images and bar codes of products, can verify products and help prevent errors in filling and dispensing drugs to patients.

Order Entry

Medication safety is further enhanced if pharmacy technicians know drug names, pharmacy terminologies, and medical jargon properly and by heart. It allows pharmacists and technicians to enter the right prescriptions. However, pharmacists and technicians often enter new drugs incorrectly because they are still unfamiliar with it. Other times, they may select something else that they're familiar with. For this reason, it's important for pharmacists and technicians to work together.

Pharmacists and technicians must be able to come up with the best method and computer systems on how they can get the latest information about new drugs and distribute this information to their patients and customers. In fact, it is the job of technicians to know and understand the different safety features of computer systems, such as drug alerts, to improve accuracy, efficiency, and medication safety.

Pharmacy technicians can receive numerous drug alerts, often prompting them to ignore it or override it through a computer system. However, it's important for technicians to always inform the pharmacist of all alerts about various clinical warnings and notifications such as duplications, allergies, interactions, and new medications. Pharmacists, on the other hand, should inform commercial or corporate software developers of redundant and unnecessary alerts. This concern should be discussed, so it can be properly turned off.

Point of Sale

Errors may still occur at the point of sale even if the prescription has been filled correctly. You may dispense medications that were not intended for a patient. It can be avoided with consistent use of second identifiers. You should be asking a customer, especially the one picking up the medications, to provide other forms of identification on behalf of the patient. You can then compare this information on the prescription vial and receipt. Reviewing prescriptions at the point of sale is the best final check you can provide.

Other internal protocols can also be adapted to. Technicians can also refer dispensing to pharmacists if a customer has ordered high-alert medications at the point of sale. If a customer or patient is new, you can use notation bags for purchased prescription drugs. Major changes in dosages and medications can also be referred to pharmacists so they can provide proper counseling to patients at the point of sale.

Pharmacy Quality Assurance_CHAPTER 6

Pharmacy Quality Assurance makes up 7.5% of the exam. Here are the knowledge areas that you need to study about under this domain:

1. Inventory control systems and quality assurance practices
2. Infection control documentation and procedures
3. Regulations and guidelines of risk management
4. Necessary communication channels to ensure appropriate problem follow-up and resolution
5. Efficiency, customer satisfaction, and productivity measures

Quality Assurance Activities

Pharmacy technicians perform quality assurance activities in pharmacies in all type of settings including the following:

- ✓ Reviewing fraud issues and billing discrepancies
- ✓ Certification, training, and education
- ✓ Coordinating errors in communication
- ✓ Inventory control
- ✓ Multiple-point checking

Quality and Safety

As part of quality assurance, pharmacy technicians develop, evaluate, and implement activities, policies, and procedures that govern pharmacy quality and safety. To do this, they are capable in the following competencies:

1: Promote the development and maintenance of a safe working environment

2: Make sure that products are of high integrity, quality, and reliable

3: Contribute to continuous risk management and quality improvement activities associated with drug distribution systems

4: Contribute to the patient safety culture

Safe Working Environment

To create a safe working environment, pharmacy technicians should be able to identify factors that affect it. Factors include ergonomics, procedural consistency, and resource allocation should be improved. Distractions in the workplace should also be managed and as much as possible, minimized.

Personal wellness is also considered a significant factor that has an impact on providing a safe working environment. It's important that pharmacy technicians have a work-life balance, are not deprived of sleep, and are emotionally and physically healthy.

Finally and more importantly, pharmacy technicians should be able to handle hazardous chemicals safely and adequately. There should be minimal exposure on the technician's part. It should also reduce environmental contamination.

Quality Products

To ensure the integrity, quality, and safety of pharmacy products, technicians are tasked to maintain the functionality and cleanliness of the dispensing, packaging, and compounding of medications. At the same time, it's important for technicians to keep storage equipment used in medicines to be functional and clean as well.

Pharmacy technicians should ensure that medications, ingredients used in compounding, and other drug-related chemicals and substances are transported, transferred, and stored under favorable conditions. A favorable condition should meet the requirements that maintain the integrity, quality, and safety of pharmacy products. One of the most widely used transfer and storage system is the cold chain management. As a pharmacy technician, you should be familiar with different types of storage systems used in pharmacies and drug-manufacturing industry.

Also, pharmacy technicians are expected to evaluate the quality of products and other pharmacy supplies. You should study about different, recognized quality assurance techniques that you will be used to inspect products. Some of the most common QA techniques include

- ✓ Identification and use of quality markers issued by manufacturers,
- ✓ Verification of supplier legitimacy, and most commonly
- ✓ Visual inspection

Risk Management and Quality Improvement

Pharmacy technicians will also be participating in activities that involve various drug distribution systems. As part of this task, you will be continuously contributing to risk management and quality improvement in different pharmacy settings. To accomplish this task, you will be:

- ✓ identifying high-risk processes, high-alert drugs, close call, and medication incidences

- ✓ responding effectively to the occurrence mentioned above to prevent reoccurrence and lessen harm,

- ✓ practicing and applying risk management principles by managing, recognizing, and anticipating situations that pose a risk to patients, and

- ✓ also applying principles quality improvement regularly.

Patient Safety Culture

To play your part in making sure that the culture of patient safety is continuously and practiced continuously, and at the same time improve it, you will be applying principles of patient safety. You will also use best practices when a medication incident occurs and inform patients about it. At the workplace, on the other hand, you will be sharing information about system changes, resolutions, problems, and lessons to the rest of your coworkers.

Medication Order Entry and Fill Process_CHAPTER 7

Medication Order Entry and Fill Process makes up 8.75% of the exam. It is divided into the following areas:

1. Order entry process
2. Data entry, intake, and interpretation
3. Calculate doses required
4. Fill process
5. Labeling requirements
6. Packaging requirements
7. Dispensing process

The Script

While filling a prescription is one of a pharmacy technician's most commonly performed duties, it is also one of the most important. Transcribing a doctor's writing into lay terms is not easy. Sometimes, it can be nearly impossible, making the life of a technician frustrating.

However, there is nothing that time and experience can't help perfect. With the right training and education, pharmacy technicians can quickly determine whether a prescription process needs the assistance of the pharmacist. Pharmacists anyway, don't always get the transcription of a prescription right – also one of the reasons how pharmacy technicians provide an extra layer of medication safety. If the pharmacist and pharmacy technician can't decipher a doctor's writing, it's the job of the technician to call the physician's office to verify and clarify a patient's prescription, also called the script.

Order Entry and Fill Process

There is a similarity in the process of reading and documenting a doctor's order whether a pharmacy technician is working in a closed-door pharmacy, community pharmacy, institutional pharmacy, or any other pharmacy setting. The following significant concepts are applied to the order entry and fill process of medications:

- ✓ Order entry process
- ✓ Calculate required doses
- ✓ Data entry, interpretation, and intake
- ✓ Requirements for labeling (e.g., patient-specific information, expiration date, auxiliary and warning labels)
- ✓ Fill method (e.g., preparing a product for the final check, measuring, applying appropriate handling requirements, selecting the right product)
- ✓ Dispensing process (e.g., distribution, documentation, validation)
- ✓ Requirements for packaging (e.g., light-resistant, child-resistant, PVC, glass, syringes, type of bags)

Processing a Prescription

While there is a difference in the order entry and fill processing of the script based on the pharmacy setting, there are five steps that are commonly required to process a prescription.

Step 1: Receiving a prescription from a patient or customer

Step 2: Deciphering the order

Step 3: Entering patient information into a database or computer system

Step 4: Dispensing the medicine

Step 5: Providing consultation to patient

The first four steps are typically assigned to pharmacy technicians. Pharmacists are given the task to provide consultation to patients. However, whoever is tasked with these steps, full concentration and focus are required. For each stage, there are several other essential tasks to accomplish and points to remember that are enumerated below.

- ✓ Exhibit the ability to prioritize filling prescriptions
- ✓ Keep in mind: the five medication safety rights of patients
    - steps to reduce medication errors
    - kinds of automated machines used to fill orders
    - the essential information required for labels and prescriptions
    - the laws that govern pharmacy technician's duties and responsibilities when dispensing medicines

- ✓ Differentiate: between outpatient and inpatient information requirements
  - filling methods used for non-controlled substances and controlled substances

Pharmacy Processing Key Points

When preparing for the Pharmacy Technician Certification Board exam, you should be focusing on these critical points that are related to pharmacy processing:

- ✓ Requirements for family members or patients picking up medication
- ✓ Requirements for filing hard copies of prescriptions
- ✓ How to properly process refills
- ✓ Who is authorized to conduct patient consultations
- ✓ The rights of patients to receive proper medication safety
- ✓ Importance of computer dispensing systems
- ✓ Importance of auxiliary labels for medications
- ✓ Instead of using childproof caps, get the required authorization to use snap-on caps
- ✓ The number of times a prescription should be checked when a pharmacy technician is filling the order
- ✓ Importance of knowing why and when to ask help from a pharmacist

- ✓ The required patient information in different types of pharmacy settings
- ✓ The differences between the information required on prescriptions for outpatients and inpatients
- ✓ Who is authorized to transfer order from one pharmacy to another
- ✓ Who is allowed to call in a prescription
- ✓ The different ways on how a medicine can be submitted for processing to a pharmacy
- ✓ The steps in prescription filling

Pharmacy Inventory Management_CHAPTER 8

The domain of Pharmacy Inventory Management makes up 8.75% of the exam. Here are the knowledge areas that you need to study about under this domain:

1. Function and application of National Drug Code (NDC), expiration dates, and lot numbers
2. Approved/preferred or formulary product list
3. Ordering and receiving processes
4. Storage requirements
5. Removal of inventory

Daily operations in the pharmacy environment involve an inventory of all medical supplies and medications. It is one of the pharmacy technician's significant responsibilities to manage inventory. The profitability of a pharmacy can be increased if a pharmacy technician conducts careful inventory management. More importantly, however, inventory management ensures that a pharmacy can serve the needs of patients and its customers with adequate stock of supplies and medications.

A pharmacy technician's level of involvement in the management of a pharmacy's inventory depends on the type of setting and facility. It can range from as simple as restocking supplies and ordering new ones in a retail environment to maintain and purchasing all the medications in a larger healthcare facility. Still, pharmacy inventory management and its general principles remain the same even though there are location-specific considerations (remember, rules and regulations vary from state to state) and varying levels of responsibilities among technicians. In the exam, you should be able to enumerate the purpose and goals of inventory management, proving your knowledge in its proper execution.

Purpose and Goals of Inventory Management

Here are the primary purpose and goals of pharmacy technicians in managing inventory for pharmacies in different types of settings:

- ✓ Help decrease the total costs in pharmacies and more extensive healthcare facilities and organization by purchasing products and supplies with the lowest price
- ✓ Prevent extra costs associated with expiration and damage of products and supplies
- ✓ Exert minimal effort and spend less time in purchasing and ordering of medications tasks
- ✓ Lower costs of drugs by ordering in bulk from wholesalers
- ✓ Decrease the maintenance cost of managing an inventory
- ✓ Prevent sudden out-of-stock occurrences to decrease the impact on patients

While these are the general purpose and goals of pharmacy inventory management, there are two main goals that pharmacy technicians should keep in mind.

First, pharmacy technicians must make sure that patients will get the right medications when they need it. Steps should be made to ensure that commonly used drugs are available for use and are stocked regularly. These medications shouldn't be damaged or outdated as well. Regularly stocked medications are based on the needs and demand of the pharmacy itself (in whatever setting), customers, and patients. Products that are difficult to acquire, costly, and rarely used meanwhile, can be ordered only when needed.

Secondly, pharmacy technicians must apply inventory management for the lowering of medication costs. There are four ways that technicians are expected to use to ensure that costs are kept at a minimum.

> **1:** Majority of pharmacies prefer to order their supplies and products from wholesalers. Other pharmacies, on the other hand, close deals with specific drug companies for contract pricing. Either of these two sources provides lower costs when purchasing medications. Pharmacy technicians can buy medicines directly from drug manufacturers or wholesalers to keep costs at a minimum that can benefit both patients and pharmacies or healthcare facilities.

> **2:** Regularly processing returns and properly managing stocks can help keep medication costs at a minimum.

> **3:** Using medications before their expiration dates can also help minimize profit loss and control medication costs.

> **4:** Another way of reducing medication costs is by using delivery systems that make acquisition efficient and reasonably priced.

Pharmacy Billing and Reimbursement_CHAPTER 9

Pharmacy Billing and Reimbursement makes up 8.75% of the exam. It is divided into the following areas:

1. Reimbursement plans and policies
2. Third-party resolution
3. Third-party reimbursement systems
4. Healthcare reimbursement systems
5. Coordination of benefits

As part of pharmacy billing and reimbursement, pharmacy technicians should be knowledgeable in private plans, CMS (Centers for Medicare & Medicaid), PPO (Preferred Provider Organization) plan, and HMOs (Health Maintenance Organizations). Familiarity with health insurance, insurance claims, medication assistance programs, and other billing and reimbursement systems is also expected from technicians.

Pharmacy Billing Cycle

Billing in most community pharmacies typically involves the following steps:

Step 1: Receiving a patient's prescription

Step 2: Important Gathering data from patient

Step 3: Entering patient data into the pharmacy database

Step 4: Pharmacy claim transmittal

Step 5: Third-party payor adjudication

Step 6: Point-of-sale

Step 7: Payment processing

Some of these steps have already been discussed in the Medication Order Entry and Fill Process. In this knowledge domain, the relations between these steps are further examined.

Receiving a Patient's Prescription

Pharmacy technicians are required to note a prescription's source, whether it is from Medicaid or Medicare healthcare, upon receiving it from a patient. Insurance companies are requesting this information, making it a common practice for technicians to track where a patient's script is from. A prescription origin code (POC) is used to track prescriptions.

Gathering Important Data from Patient

The following information is required from a patient:

- ✓ Disease, illness, or any medical condition
- ✓ Personal information including
    - correct full name

- date of birth
- contact information, and
- home address

✓ Any form of allergy

✓ Medication insurance information including
  - member number
  - group number
  - bank identification number (BIN)
  - insurance name, and most importantly,
  - coverage type (e.g., primary, secondary)

The pharmacy technician verifies all this information.

Data Entry

After gathering the necessary information, the pharmacy technician will have to enter the data into the software management system that the pharmacy uses. This moves the process of prescription forward. Typically, the following data are registered:

✓ **Prescriber information** – includes the doctor's or licensed medical practitioner's information

✓ **Prescription information** – consists of the doctor's or licensed medical practitioner's recommended medications or medical supplies

- ✓ **DAW codes** – includes dispense as written (DAW) codes which refer to product selection recommended by doctors or licensed medical practitioners. Systems used are:

Code	Value
0	Product selection not indicated (missing values may occur)
1	Prescriber disallows substitution
2	Substitution allowed - patient requests branded product
3	Substitution allowed - pharmacist selected product
4	Substitution allowed - generic drug not available
5	Substitution allowed - brand drug substituted for a generic drug
6	Override
7	Substitution not allowed - brand drug mandated by law
8	Substitution allowed - generic drug not available in the market
9	Other

- ✓ **Drug information** – includes the drug's name, manufacturer, and NDC (National Drug Code)
- ✓ **Third-party payor** – includes insurance, medical plans, HMOs, and other third-party reimbursement systems
- ✓ **Patient information** – consists of the patient's personal information and medical conditions

Pharmacy Claim Transmittal

The pharmacy claim transmittal is the pathway followed for claiming third-party reimbursements. It is processed exclusively through pharmacy management software. It is at this point that a pharmacy prepares the transmittal of a prescription to a third-party payor to verify a patient's medical insurance or plan. If confirmed, the purchase of prescribed drugs is approved. Some of the common reasons why claims are disapproved include:

- ✓ The incorrect or incomplete entry of doctor's or licensed medical practitioner's information
- ✓ The inaccurate or incomplete entry of patient's insurance information
- ✓ Inactive insurance
- ✓ Invalid quantity, wrong supply, or early refill of medications
- ✓ Unauthorized or non-covered drugs

In the case that a prescription is not approved for reimbursement, it is the duty of the doctor or patient to call the third-party payor or its pharmacy benefits manager (PBM) to obtain approval. If a patient has more than one medical insurance plans, split-billing and coordination of benefits are applied.

Third-Party Payor Adjudication

This electronic process, also called real-time claim adjudication (RTCA), is accomplished in a matter of seconds. A claim is adjudicated once the prescription is accepted. This means that the payor determines the actual cost that a patient has to pay and the financial responsibility of the patient's insurance plan. It is done by comparing the actual charges with the coverage of a patient's benefits plan.

Point-of-Sale

While medications can be reimbursed, additional payments may still be charged from patients when medications are picked up. Deductibles, copays, and unauthorized or non-covered medications are paid by patients. Pharmacy technicians, while assigned to point-of-sale tasks, can accept various payment options including debit cards, credit cards, checks, manufacturer coupons, and cash. Payment information is also included in data entry in pharmacy management systems.

Payment Processing

On the other hand, pharmacy technicians will have to take care of payment processing from insurance companies. Typically, companies send out an RA (remittance advice) every 30 to 60 days to pharmacies. This advice provides details about the patient claims that the companies will have to pay to the pharmacies where patients purchased their medications. Along with the RA, also called the explanation of benefits, insurance companies send their payments for all the prescription processed by a pharmacy for a particular period of time.

Other Reimbursement Methods

Aside from third-party payor reimbursements, pharmacies also accept other methods such as the two below. These methods are commonly used in home infusion, long-term healthcare, and home healthcare settings.

Episode-of-Care Reimbursement

In this type of reimbursement method, pharmacies pay a lump sum to insurance companies and third-party payors for all the provided services related to a single disease or condition. This means that payment and reimbursement depend on the episode and not the service provided. It's a method that eliminates individual charges and fees, which makes sense for longer, expected healthcare. It's a suitable payment method that controls costs systematically. Meanwhile, the cost contracted with a pharmacy under this reimbursement method is called the capitation fee.

Fee-for-Service Reimbursement

Fee-for-service, on the other hand, is the exact opposite of the episode-of-care reimbursement method. A set price is paid for all the types of services provided by healthcare facilities. Insurance companies, on the other hand, pay the healthcare facilities for every single service covered by a patient's plan. Collectively, fees paid by insurance companies are called charges in healthcare.

Claims by patients are forwarded to the third-party payor. The insurance company then sends out payments to healthcare facilities.

Pharmacy Information System Usage and Application_CHAPTER 10

The last knowledge domain that you have to study for the Pharmacy Technician Certification Exam is the Pharmacy Information System Usage and Application. Its weight in the test is equivalent to 10%, which is relatively more compared to the last three knowledge domains of the exam — the reasons why software companies developing pharmacy management software hire pharmacy technicians among their team.

Knowledge areas for this part of the test include:

1. Computer applications for pharmacy-related tasks especially for the documentation of the dispensing of medication orders or prescriptions

2. Documentation management, pharmacy computer applications, and databases

Pharmacy technicians are entrusted with a number of functions and operations that rely upon strict policies and procedures. To accomplish these functions and operations, and adhere to its established rules, technicians are expected to know how to use computer systems. Aside from holding a pharmacy's database, computer systems play a huge role in delivering efficient operations in pharmacies, further emphasizing the importance of technicians' knowledge in this area.

Pharmacy technicians should have a basic knowledge of computer applications and terminologies. As a technician, you should also be familiar with the pharmacist's different and the roles and responsibilities in using computer-based systems as well. Both you and the pharmacist will be focusing on the multiple operations that can contribute to the effective and safe practices of prescribing, administering, distributing, and dispensing or pharmaceuticals, medical devices, equipment, and supplies.

In general, the following software is used in different pharmacy settings.

Pharmacy Interfaces

At the center of it all, the software that glues the pieces together is the pharmacy interface. Aside from receiving new prescriptions, it enables pharmacists and technicians to send and receive requests for renewal of prescriptions from doctors who are connected to the interface. Everything works electronically and is mostly automated.

There are two interface workflows used in pharmacies. Pharmacies choose between these workflows depending on how the operation of a pharmacy is managed.

> **Pharmacy-centric:** preferred workflow in pharmacies. They enter prescription orders into the system, which automates updates for patients' medical records.

> **Facility-centric:** preferred workflow by insurance companies. Healthcare facilities enter prescription orders directly into patients' electronic medical records, and then automatically sent to the pharmacy.

While the majority of the insurance providers prefer the facility-centric interface, it doesn't mean that it is better than the pharmacy-centric interface. They like it better because of their ability to control medication orders and medical records.

Pharmacy Computer Applications

Computer applications present a list of applications accepted as part of pharmacy computer systems. They should meet minimum qualifications including the ability to:

- ✓ Automate labor-intensive activities used to support services related to drug distribution
- ✓ Automate label product which is used to generate unit dose cart fill list and manual backup profile
- ✓ Automatically include the description and scope of information for unit and IV dose labels
- ✓ Include crediting and charging functions
- ✓ Include free-form capabilities

Some of the most commonly sought-after computer applications include:

- ✓ data confidentiality
- ✓ drug interaction flagging
- ✓ medication profiling
- ✓ documentation management
- ✓ reports
    - hard copy reports
    - census report
    - inventory report

- usage reports
- override reports
- diversion reports

✓ databases
- pharmacy databases
- drug databases

Practice Test_CHAPTER 11

This practice test can help you understand what can be expected of the Pharmacy Technician Certification Exam. There are 30 items in this test. Answers are given to the end of the training test, so you can review your answers and where you got it wrong.

To help you simulate the exam environment, time yourself as you answer these questions. The allotted time for the 80 items in the official exam is 50 minutes. If you can do better than that, then you sure are ready for the certification exam.

Good luck!

Questions

1. A medication order refers to a

   A. Medications ordered through the phone or transcribed through a system
   B. Script
   C. Written prescription
   D. Drugs ordered by a doctor for a patient

2. Which one is not used to treat epilepsy?

   A. Gabapentin
   B. Lovastatin
   C. Valproic acid
   D. Diazepam

3. What is the difference between a suspension and a solution?

    A ☐ A solution has large particles, while a suspension has smaller ones
    B ☐ A solution has small particles, while a suspension has larger ones
    C ☐ A suspension is homogenous, while a solution is not
    D ☐ None of the above

4. Which law formed the US Food and Drug Administration (FDA)?

    A ☐ Durham-Humphrey Act of 1951
    B ☐ Food, Drugs, and Cosmetics Act of 1938 (FDCA)
    C ☐ Kefauver-Harris Amendment of 1962
    D ☐ Health Act of 1970 (OSHA)

5. Preventive medical services covered by many health plans include:

    A ☐ Pediatric and adolescent immunizations
    B ☐ Annual physical examinations
    C ☐ Prenatal care
    D ☐ All of the above

6. Calculate the cost of 30 tablets of Metformin if the cost for 100 tablets is $140.00 and the percentage markup on the prescription is a 5?

    A ☐ $14.07
    B ☐ $45.83
    C ☐ $1.04

D ☐ $44.1

7. Each one below serves as a purpose of pharmacy inventory management except one.

A ☐ Increase costs to boost income by ordering medications from wholesalers.
B ☐ Decrease total costs by focusing on purchasing products at the lowest cost.
C ☐ Prevent costs associated with the expiration and damage of inventory.
D ☐ Minimize the occurrence of unexpected out-of-stocks

8. Non-sterile compounded product labels include the following except:

A ☐ Storage conditions
B ☐ The concentration of active ingredients in the final compounded product
C ☐ Expiration date
D ☐ The compounded product's internal control number

9. DX stands for

A ☐ Prescription
B ☐ Symptoms
C ☐ Diagnosis
D ☐ Prognosis

10. The listing of approved drugs that are available for use.

A ☐ Database
B ☐ Drugs report
C ☐ Medications database
D ☐ Formulary

11. The number that is assigned by manufacturers to the drugs they produce. It can be seen on prescription stock packages.

    A ☐ Lot number
    B ☐ Dosage form
    C ☐ NDC
    D ☐ DAW code

12. How many ccs of syrup should be dispensed for a 15-day supply of Valproic acid syrup if a patient needs to take 750mg in the morning and 1000mg in the evening?

    A ☐ 500cc
    B ☐ 515cc
    C ☐ 520cc
    D ☐ 525cc

13. Prohibits mail order prescription drugs in a prescription drug plan unless a non-mail order prescription drug is covered.

    A ☐ Prescription Drug Equity Law
    B ☐ Combat Methamphetamine Epidemic Act of 2005
    C ☐ USP 797
    D ☐ Freedom of Choice Law

14. The step in the pharmacy billing cycle that allows electronic data interchange.

    A ☐ Payor adjudication
    B ☐ Pharmacy claim transmittal
    C ☐ Payment processing

D ☐ Follow-up of accounts receivable

15. One of these drugs is an antihistamine.

    A ☐ Lisinopril
    B ☐ Glucophage
    C ☐ Simvastatin
    D ☐ Cetirizine

16. In compliance with the HIPAA, pharmacies must provide new patients with what?

    A ☐ Patient privacy policy
    B ☐ Patient counseling
    C ☐ Preventive medical screening
    D ☐ Medication order

17. The number that indicates the batch number of a drug produced by a drug manufacturer

    A ☐ NDC
    B ☐ SIG Code
    C ☐ Lot number
    D ☐ RTS

18. 30ml is equivalent to:

    A ☐ One tablespoon
    B ☐ 1 ounce
    C ☐ Two teaspoon
    D ☐ 10cc

19. What is referred to as inappropriate medication use?

- A ☐ Medication error
- B ☐ Drug dependency
- C ☐ Medication safety
- D ☐ None of the above

20. Which organization tracks medication errors aside from the FDA?

- A ☐ CDC
- B ☐ NRDC
- C ☐ Institute for Safe Medication Practices
- D ☐ EOC

21. Which agency did the Comprehensive Drugs Abuse Prevention and Control Act of 1970 helped create?

- A ☐ Federal Bureau of Investigation (FBI)
- B ☐ National Institutes of Health (NIH)
- C ☐ Healthcare Infection Control Practices Advisory Committee
- D ☐ Drugs Enforcement Administration (DEA)

22. Which is a brand name for Omeprazole?

- A ☐ Ventolin®
- B ☐ Depakote®
- C ☐ Prilosec®
- D ☐ Soma®

23. How is insulin administered to a patient?

- A ☐ Injection

B		Oral administration
C		Intravenous
D		Suppository

24. What is the route of administration?

A		The US government's plans and programs
B		The marketing and sales strategy of a pharmacy
C		The Department of Health and Human Services' organizational chart
D		The different methods of taking medications

25. In the pharmacy billing cycle, what is the last process that a pharmacy technician has to do?

A		Payment processing
B		Collections
C		Patient interview
D		Payor adjudication

26. A patient has a prescription order for 10ml of medication, twice a day for seven days. How much medication does the patient need to order to fill the doctor's 7-day requirement? Convert your answer to ounces.

A		2oz
B		3.5oz
C		5ml
D		5oz

27. What is the recall level for medications that have been considered harmful to the patient's health?

   A ☐ Class I recall
   B ☐ Class II recall
   C ☐ Class III recall
   D ☐ Class IV recall

28. What is a stand-alone computer system that manages data accessed from a database and runs software programs

   A ☐ Clinical Decision Support Systems (CDSS)
   B ☐ Minicomputers
   C ☐ Microcomputers or Personal Computers (PCs)
   D ☐ Ambulatory Pharmacy Computer Functions

29. Microcomputers or personal computers are used in pharmacies for the following functions except one:

   A ☐ Workload statistics
   B ☐ Non-formulating drug use
   C ☐ Adverse drug reporting
   D ☐ Filling a prescription

30. Remittance advice is also called.

   A ☐ Explanation of benefits
   B ☐ Pharmacy claim
   C ☐ Formulary
   D ☐ Electronic data interchange

Answers

1. A

A medication order is a written request by a doctor or licensed medical practitioner (both are also called the prescriber). It used to order medications or drugs from pharmacies in an inpatient setting. It is different from a prescription, which is for an outpatient setting or ambulatory care.

2. B

Mevacor (Lovastatin) is not indicated for epilepsy treatment. It is used for the treatment of elevated lipid levels.

3. B

A solution is a "homogenous" mixture where two or more liquids or solids are combined. It is homogenous because particles of the different liquids or solids are too small to be differentiated apart. In a suspension, the particles are larger. They repel each other, making liquids and solids settle out or separate over time. This makes it important to shake any suspension before taking it.

4. B

The US Food and Drug Administration's (FDA) history dates back to as early as the late 1880s. However, it was President Franklin Roosevelt's Food, Drugs, and Cosmetics Act of 1938 (FDCA) that paved the way for the FDA to gain more authority over the distribution and manufacturing of pharmaceuticals. The law helped FDA required applications to be filed by drug manufacturers before they can create new drugs.

5. D

The US Department of Health preventive medical services covered by various health plans is categorized into three sets: for adults, women, and children. For each set, services include:

Adults	Women	Children
Abdominal aortic aneurysm one-time screening	For pregnant women: Anemia screening Breastfeeding comprehensive support and counseling Contraception	Alcohol and drug use assessments Autism screening Behavioral assessments Blood pressure screening
Alcohol misuse screening and counseling		
Aspirin use	Folic acid supplements	Cervical dysplasia screening
Blood pressure screening	Gestational diabetes screening	Depression screening Developmental screening
Cholesterol screening	Gonorrhea screening	Dyslipidemia screening
Colorectal cancer screening	Hepatitis B screening Rh Incompatibility screening	Fluoride chemoprevention supplements
Depression screening		Gonorrhea preventive medication
Diabetes (Type 2) screening	Syphilis screening Expanded tobacco intervention and counseling	Hearing screening
Diet counseling		Body mass index (BMI) measurements
Hepatitis B screening		
Hepatitis C screening	Urinary tract or other infection screening	Hematocrit or hemoglobin screening
HIV screening		
Immunization vaccines for:		Hemoglobinopathies or sickle cell screening
Diphtheria	For women in general: Breast cancer genetic test counseling (BRCA)	
Hepatitis A		Hepatitis B screening
Hepatitis B	Breast cancer mammography screenings	HIV screening
Human Papillomavirus (HPV)		Hypothyroidism screening Immunization vaccines including:
Herpes Zoster	Breast cancer chemoprevention counseling	Diphtheria, Tetanus, Pertussis (Whooping Cough)
Influenza (flu shot)		
Measles		
Meningococcal	Cervical cancer screening	Haemophilus influenza type b
Mumps		
Pneumococcal	Chlamydia infection screening	Hepatitis A
Pertussis		Hepatitis B
Rubella	Domestic and interpersonal violence	Human Papillomavirus (PVU)
Tetanus		

Varicella (Chickenpox) Lung cancer screening Obesity screening and counseling Sexually transmitted infection (STI) prevention counseling Syphilis screening Tobacco Use screening	screening and counseling Gonorrhea screening HIV screening and counseling Human Papillomavirus (HPV) DNA test Osteoporosis screening Rh incompatibility screening Sexually transmitted infections counseling Syphilis screening Tobacco use screening and interventions Well-woman visits	Inactivated Poliovirus Measles Influenza (flu shot) Meningococcal Rotavirus Varicella (Chickenpox) Pneumococcal Iron supplements Lead screening Medical history for all children Obesity screening and counseling Oral health risk assessment Phenylketonuria (PKU) screening Sexually transmitted infection (STI) Tuberculin testing Vision screening

6. D

The cost for 100 tablets of Metformin is $140; therefore, the cost for a single tablet of Olanzapine should be $140/100 = $1.40.

The % mark-up on a prescription is 5.

Cost for Metformin	Mark-up on Rx
$140	$5
$1.40	?

5 x 1.40 / 100 = $0.07, therefore a dispensing cost of each tablet of Metformin should be $1.40 + $0.07 = $1.47.

The cost for dispensing 30 tablets should be $4.83 x 30 = $44.1.

7. A

The purpose of inventory management in pharmacies include:

- Help decrease the total costs in pharmacies and larger healthcare facilities and organization by purchasing products and supplies with the lowest cost
- Prevent extra costs associated with expiration and damage of products and supplies
- Exert minimal effort and spend less time in purchasing and ordering of medications tasks
- Lower costs of medications by ordering in bulk from wholesalers
- Decrease the maintenance cost of managing an inventory
- Prevent sudden out-of-stock occurrences to decrease the impact on patients

8. D

Product labels follow all state and federal requirements. Labels of compounded products include, but not limited to:

- List of active ingredients;
- The concentration of active ingredients;
- A lot number of the compounded product;
- Estimated best before date or expiry date of the compound; and
- Storage instructions

Medications packaged individually should be individually labeled with the name of the compound, expiry date, and lot number. It is placed in a larger container with a prescription label for dispensing.

9. C

Rx stands for a prescription. Sx stands for symptoms. Dx, or dx, stands for diagnosis.

10. D

A formulary is a list of drugs approved by the FDA and therefore, can be prescribed by doctors and licensed medical practitioners to patients.

11. C

The National Drug Code (NDC) number is an 11-digit number assigned to drugs

The Drug Listing Act of 1972 requires drug manufacturers to provide FDA with a list of drugs they have created, compounded, prepared, or processed before making them commercially available. Drugs and other drug-related products are assigned with a National Drug Code (NDC), a unique, 11-digit, 3-segmented number. This number is used to identify each commercial drug in the US. The FDA lists and updates all NDC in the NDC Directory.

12. A

Many insurance providers and pharmacy benefits management (PBM) companies promoted the use of mail-order prescription drugs in the US. However, the government noticed that the top providers and PBM companies managed their own mail-order pharmacies, which was the reason why these companies promoted mail-order prescriptions. The Prescription Drug Equity Law, or the Prescription Drug Benefit Equity Act of 2006, was created to allow patients to purchase their prescription drugs from any pharmacy that they prefer.

13. B

The pharmacy claim transmittal is the pathway followed for claiming third-party reimbursements. It is processed exclusively through pharmacy management software. It is at this point that a pharmacy processes the transmittal of a prescription to a third-party payor to verify a patient's medical insurance or plan. If verified, the purchase of prescribed drugs is approved.

14. D

Antihistamines are used to treat allergies and other related symptoms. These are some of the best-known antihistamines available:

Prescription	Over-the-Counter
Xyzal (Levocabastine oral)	Alavert, Claritin (Loratadine)
Livostin (Levocabastine eyedrops)	Allegra (Fexofenadine)
Atarax, Vistaril (Hydroxyzine)	Benadryl (Diphenhydramine)
Emadine (Emedastine eyedrops)	Tavist (Clemastine)
Clarinex (Desloratadine)	Dimetane (Brompheniramine)
Cyproheptadine	Zyrtec (Cetirizine)
Palgic (Carbinoxamine)	Chlor-Trimeton (Chlorpheniramine)
Astelin, Astepro (Azelastine nasal sprays)	
Optivar (Azelastine eyedrops)	

15. A

Accountability Act (HIPAA) of 1996 provides security provisions and data privacy to keep medical information safe and confidential.

16. C

    A lot number is part of the FDA's requirement for drug manufacturers to provide. It is vital in product tracing information and promotes drug quality and security in the case of a recall or corrections.

17. B

    30ml = 1 ounce

    1ml = 0.033814

    30 x 0.033814 = 1.01442

    Round off answer = 1

18. A

    According to the National Coordinating Council for Medication Error Reporting and Prevention (NCCMERP), a medication error is a medical event that could have been prevented. Otherwise, it will cause harm to patients or lead to inappropriate use of medications. Medication errors are not exclusive to patients only. It can also be committed by healthcare professionals. The Council emphasizes that errors can also occur during the monitoring, education, administration, distribution, dispensing, compounding, packaging, labeling, order communication, and prescribing of drugs.

19. C

    Patients, consumers, and healthcare professionals can report medication errors to the Institute for Safe

Medication Practices, a non-profit organization based in Philadelphia. They publish a consumer newsletter called Safe Medicine, which focuses on medication errors.

20. D

The Drug Enforcement Administration was created by the Comprehensive Drugs Abuse Prevention and Control Act of 1970. Under the US Department of Justice, it combats drug use and smuggling in the USA.

21. C

Prilosec® is one of the top-selling Omeprazole drugs in the US. Omeprazole is a proton-pump inhibitor, which means that it is an anti-ulcer drug. It lessens the stomach's gastric acid production.

Ventolin® is an asthma medication. Depakote® is an anti-seizure drug that is also used to relieve symptoms caused by manic depression (or bipolar disorder) and headaches caused by migraine. Soma® is a muscle relaxant and is typically used to treat conditions of the skeletal muscles.

22. A

Insulin is administered through injection because it can't tolerate gastric acid in the digestive system. In an emergency or hospital settings, insulin is administered intravenously, or it is injected into the IV fluid.

Oral administration of drugs means that medications are taken by mouth. A suppository, on the other hand, is a drug that is inserted beyond the muscular sphincter in the rectum.

23. D

Route of administration is the method of how a medication is applied or taken into the body. The most routes of administration include:

- ✓ Oral – through the mouth
- ✓ Topical – on the skin
- ✓ Sublingual – under the tongue
- ✓ Inhalation – through the nose
- ✓ Injection – through blood veins. There are four types:
  - intradermal (ID),
  - subcutaneous (SC),
  - intramuscular (IM), and
  - intravenous (IV).

24. B

There are five major steps in prescription processing, but the billing cycle involves ten steps:

▶ Step 1: receipt of a prescription
▶ Step 2: patient interview
▶ Step 3: filling of a prescription
▶ Step 4: pharmacy claim transmittal
▶ Step 5: payer adjudication
▶ Step 6: point-of-sale patient payment
▶ Step 7: calculation of payer claim balance
▶ Step 8: accounts receivable follow-up
▶ Step 9: payment processing
▶ Step 10: collections and problem resolution

25. B

There are five major steps in prescription processing, but the billing cycle involves ten steps:

- Step 1: receipt of a prescription
- Step 2: patient interview
- Step 3: filling of a prescription
- Step 4: pharmacy claim transmittal
- Step 5: payer adjudication
- Step 6: point-of-sale patient payment
- Step 7: calculation of payer claim balance
- Step 8: accounts receivable follow-up
- Step 9: payment processing
- Step 10: collections and problem resolution

26. D

10ml per dose x 2 doses per day x 7 days = 140ml

30ml = 1oz

140ml / 30ml = 4.67

Round off answer = 5oz

27. A

A recall is when a manufacturer discovers that there is a correction for medication or it has to be removed from the market. It is categorized in the following classes:

- ✓ Class I: medication is recalled because it will cause serious health consequences or death.

- ✓ Class II: medication is recalled because it may cause temporary adverse health consequences or its adverse effects may happen remotely.

- ✓ Class III recall: medication is recalled because it may cause side effects, but not seriously

- ✓ Market withdrawal: medication is withdrawn from the market because it has a minor violation with the FDA.

- ✓ Medical device safety alert: medical device is most likely recalled because it may cause harm to its user.

28. C

29. D

Microcomputers include a central processing unit (CPU), monitor, and printer. It is used in the pharmacy for workload statistics, non-formulating drug use, adverse drug reporting, drug utilization evaluations, drug information, and quality assurance.

30. A

Pharmacy technicians will have to take care of payment processing from insurance companies. Typically, companies send out an RA (remittance advice) every 30 to 60 days to pharmacies. This advice provides details about the patient claims that the companies will have to pay to the pharmacies where patients purchased their medications. It is also called the explanation of benefits.

Conclusion

Thank you again for downloading this book!

I hope this eBook has helped you to prepare for the Pharmacy Technician Certification Exam. Before I go, I want to leave you some tips:

- ✓ You can search for more free practice tests online.

- ✓ Focus on what's only expected from the exam. Don't study subjects or topics that are not included in the exam's blueprint.

- ✓ The night before the exam, make sure to get enough sleep.

- ✓ Don't be late for the exam. If you have extra time between your arrival and the test, you won't be too stressed or pressured.

- ✓ Most importantly, have a positive mindset. You've done your best to study and prepare; now it's time to believe in what you can do.

Made in the USA
Middletown, DE
08 June 2019